CLOVES

MARIAN KIM

CONTENTS

MARIAN KIM

1

PROPERTIES

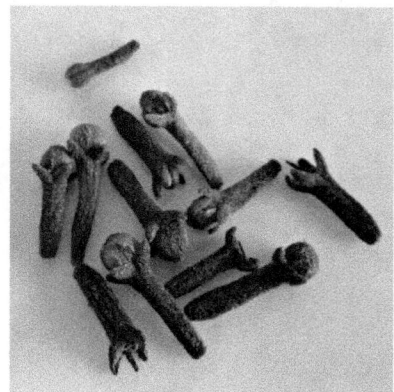

Scientific name: Syzygium aromaticum

Other names: Ding xiang, Eugenia aromatic, Caryophyllum

Nutrients: : Vitamins A, B1 (thiamine), B2 (riboflavin), B6 (pyridoxine), C and K. They also contain minerals like calcium, iron, magnesium and manganese. Cloves also contain dietary fiber.

Properties

Oil of clove contains a high concentration of eugenol which has pain relieving properties, anti-microbial properties and anti-inflammatory properties.

Cloves also have:

Antiseptic (antiviral, antibacterial, antifungal) properties

Anti-oxidant properties which protect the cells from free radical damage

Anti-aging properties

Anti-cancer properties

Rubefacient (warming and soothing) properties

Carminative (antiflatulent) properties

* * * * *

2

USES

Cold sore treatment

Cloves have been shown to hasten the healing of cold sores.

Tooth pain relief

Cloves relieve tooth pain and they are applied directly to the gum.

Mouth inflammation

Cloves can be chewed to reduce pain and swelling in inflamed mouths and throats.

Sorethroat treatment

Clove tinctures can be used as a gargle for sorethroats.

Diabetes treatment

Cloves can help manage diabetes since some of their compounds seem to improve insulin function. The help the body lower blood sugar levels by utilizing insulin more effectively.

Arthritis treatment

Clove poultice are used to treat arthritis and joint pains. The whole cloves can also be added to the bath water.

Muscle pain treatment

Clove poultices are used to treat muscle pains. The whole cloves can also be added to the bath water.

Flatulence treatment

Clove decoctions are used to treat flatulence (intestinal gas).

Indigestion treatment

Clove decoctions are used to treat indigestion since the spice is thought to stimulate the production of gastric enzymes.

Upset stomach treatment

Cloves are used to treat upset stomachs.

Coughs

Clove tea is used for productive coughs because they act as an expectorant. Cloves are also used for colds and the flu due to their analgesic and antiseptic properties.

Asthma treatment

Cloves have been used for asthma treatment.

Nausea and vomiting

Cloves are used for nausea and vomiting.

Hiccup relief

Cloves are used to treat hiccups.

Sunburn relief

Cloves are used on sunburns.

Poison ivy relief

Cloves are used for poison ivy.

Acne treatment

Cloves are used for acne treatment.

Weight loss

Cloves are used for weight loss.

Aphrodisiac

Cloves can be used as aphrodisiacs to prevent premature ejaculation.

Antihelminthic

Cloves are used to treat intestinal worms since they are thought to have anti-parasitic activity.

Stress management

Cloves are used for stress management since they can stimulate the mind and relieve mental fatigue and exhaustion. Clove oil is also used to treat depression.

Headache treatment

Cloves are used to treat headaches. Clove oil can be mixed with salt and applied to the forehead to relieve headaches.

Insect bite treatment

Cloves are used on insect bites due to their analgesic (pain relieving properties) and antiseptic properties.

Insect repellent

Cloves are effective insect repellent. Clove oil is especially beneficial for repelling mosquitos.

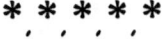

3

SAFETY PRECAUTIONS

1. Children should not take clove oil by mouth since it can cause liver damage and seizures.

2. Repeated applications of clove oil to the mouth can damage the gums, teeth and mucous membranes.

3. Persons with bleeding disorders should not take clove oil since it contains eugenol which can slow the clotting of blood.

4. Persons scheduled to have surgery should stop using cloves 2 weeks before the operation since it can potentially cause bleeding during or after surgery.

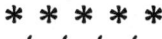

4

DRUG INTERACTIONS

1. Cloves can interact with some medications and increase bleeding since it can slow clotting of blood. Examples of these medications include:

a. Antiplatelet medications like aspirin, clopidogrel (Plavix)

b. Non-steroidal anti-inflammatory drugs (NSAIDS) like diclofenac (Voltaren), ibuprofen (Advil), naproxen (Naprosyn)

c. Anticoagulants like dalteparin (Fragmin), enoxaparin (Lovenox), heparin, Coumadin (warfarin)

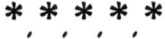

5

COOKING TIPS

Flavor: Aromatically sweet

Goes well with: Rice dishes e.g. pilau, spicy tea and coffee

Can be substituted with: Allspice, cinnamon, nutmeg

* * * * *

6

HERBAL RECIPES

Clove Tea

Equipment
Kettle

Tea cup

***

Ingredients
1 teaspoon of cloves

1 cup of boiling water

Honey to taste (optional)

***

Instructions

1. Put the cloves in a tea cup, add the boiling water and let it steep while covered for 10 -15 minutes.

2. Add honey (if using) to suit your taste before drinking.

*****

Clove Syrup

Equipment

Saucepan

Jar with airtight lid

***

Ingredients

1 quart (1000 ml) filtered water

1 cup cloves

1 cup honey

***

Instructions

1. Place the water and cloves in a saucepan and bring to a boil.

2. Reduce the heat and let it simmer while it is partially covered until the volume is reduced to half the original volume.

3. Strain the mixture through a sieve or cheesecloth to remove the cloves.

4. Measure 1 pint (500 mls) of the liquid and add the honey.

5. Cook for a few minutes as you stir it so that it thickens.

6. Store the syrup in an airtight container in the fridge for up to 2 months.

*****

Clove Poultice

Equipment

Cheesecloth or old cotton sheet strips

***

Ingredients

1 tablespoon clove powder

Boiling water

***

Instructions

1. Add enough boiling water to the cloves to form a thick paste.

2. Spoon the clove paste onto the cheesecloth (or bed sheet strips) to make the poultice.

3. To use, apply the poultice to the affected area and cover with another piece of hot, wet cloth. Replace the hot, wet cloth when it cools with another hot one to keep the poultice hot.

*****

Clove Decoction

Equipment
Non-reactive heavy saucepan

***

Ingredients
1 oz (30 grams) cloves

1 pint (500 ml) water

***

Instructions
1. Place the cloves and water in the saucepan, cover them and slowly bring the mixture to a simmering boil for 20 minutes.

2. Remove from the heat source and let the mixture cool to drinking temperature.

3. Strain the mixture, measure it and pour the liquid into a clean saucepan.

4. Heat the liquid until it begins to steam. Reduce the heat and let the liquid continue to steam until it is reduced to half its original volume. This may take 45 minutes to 1 hour.

5. Pour the decoction into a clean bottle.

***

Tips
1. Store the decoction in the refrigerator to lengthen its life.

*****

Clove Tincture

Equipment

Glass jar with tight fitting lid

Dark tincture bottles

Cheesecloth

Labels

***

Ingredients

7 oz (200 gm) of cloves

30 oz (1 liter) of 80-100 proof vodka

***

Instructions

1. Fill 1/3 of the glass jar with the cloves.

2. Add the vodka to completely fill the jar to the top.

3. Seal the jar and label it with the date of preparation and name of herb used. Store the glass jar in a dark place for 6 weeks ensuring that you shake them weekly.

4. After 6 weeks strain out the cloves with a cheesecloth and pour the tincture into dark tincture bottles.

5. Label the tincture bottles with the date and name of spice used.

6. Store your clove tinctures away from light and heat.

*****

Clove Infused Oil

Equipment

Double boiler

Large glass bowl

Sieve and cheesecloth

Sterilized dark jars

***

Ingredients

16 fl oz. (500 ml) vegetable oil like sweet almond or sunflower oil

8 oz. (250 grams) bruised cloves

***

Instructions

1. Place the cloves and oil in the glass bowl ensuring that the oil covers the cloves. Simmer them in a double boiler for 1 hour at around 120 degrees Fahrenheit (49 degrees Celsius). Do not let the mixture boil. You can repeat this step after letting the oils cool to create more concentrated clove infused oils.

2. Strain the mixture through the sieve and cheesecloth into a clean, dark jar ensuring you squeeze out as much oil as you can from the cheesecloth.

3. Label your jars with the manufacturing date, expiry date, spice and oils used. Store your clove infused oils in a cool dark place or in the refrigerator and use them within 3 months.

*****

Clove Salve

Equipment
Double boiler

Large glass bowl

Sterilized dark jars or tins

***

Ingredients
8 oz. (250 ml or 1 cup) clove infused vegetable oil (see previous recipe)

1 oz. (30 grams) beeswax

50 drops (2.5 ml or ½ teaspoon) essential oils like lavender essential oil (optional natural fragrance)

***

Instructions
1. Place the beeswax and clove infused oil in the glass bowl and melt them in a double boiler.

2. Once melted remove from the heat source, allow to cool and add the essential oils (if using).

3. Pour the melted oils into the storage jars or tins and allow to cool completely.

4. Store the salves in a cool dark place.

***

Tip
If you want softer salves you can use less beeswax – for example ¾ oz of beeswax for 1 cup of vegetable oils.

CLOVES

###

ABOUT THE AUTHOR

Marian Kim is an experienced alternative medicine practitioner.

*****

OTHER BOOKS BY THE AUTHOR

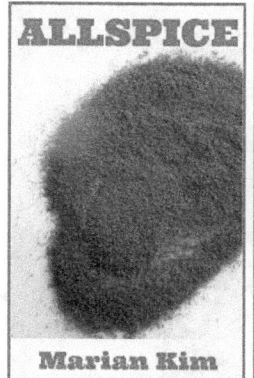

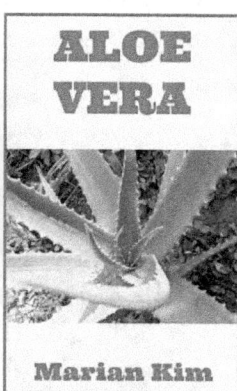

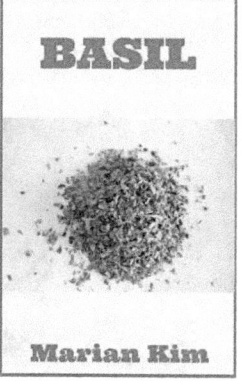

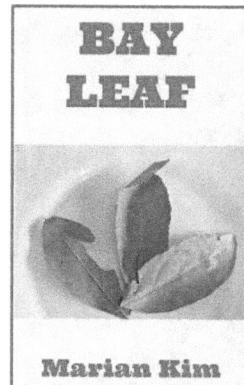

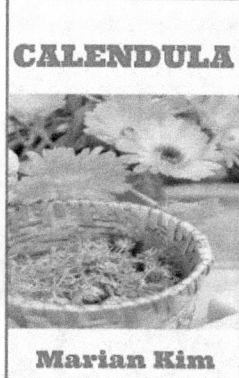

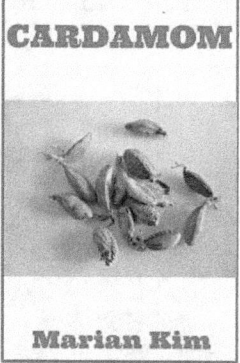

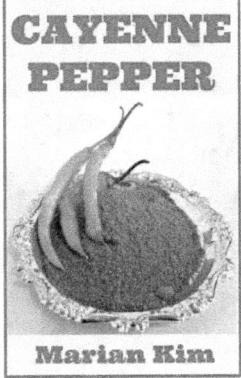

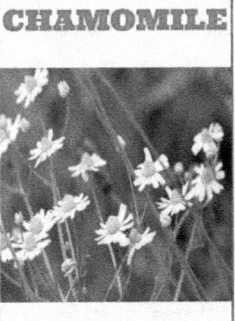

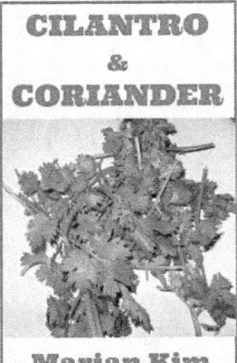

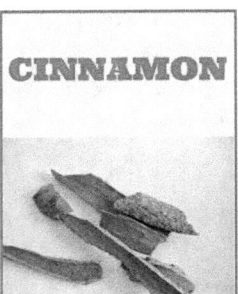

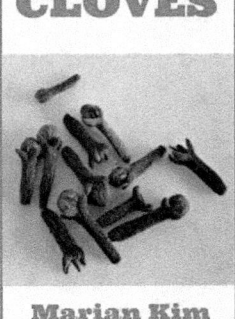

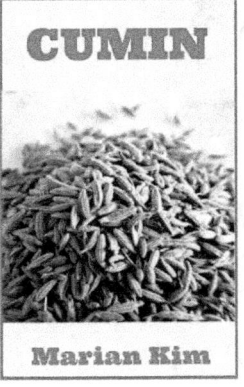

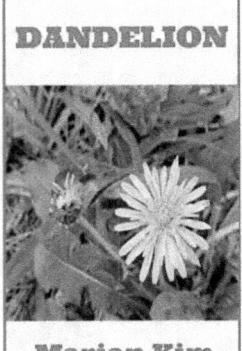

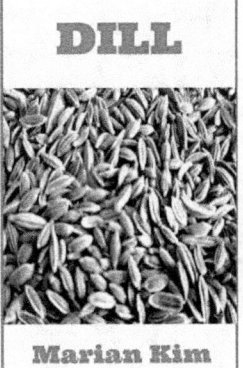

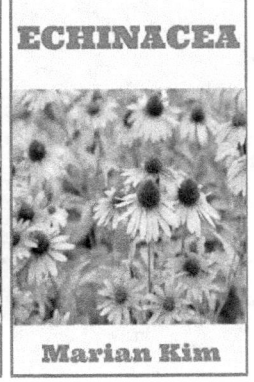

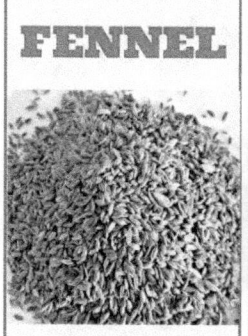

FENNEL

Marian Kim

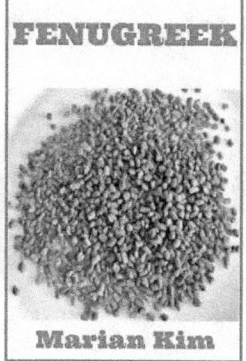

FENUGREEK

Marian Kim

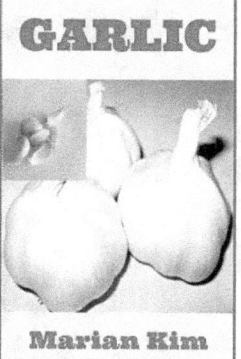

GARLIC

Marian Kim

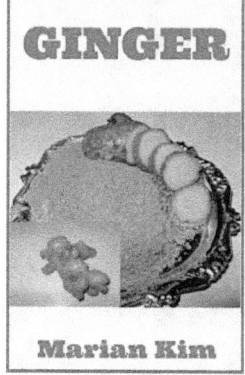

GINGER

Marian Kim

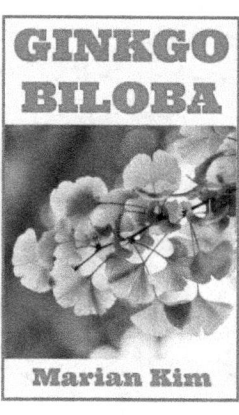

GINKGO BILOBA

Marian Kim

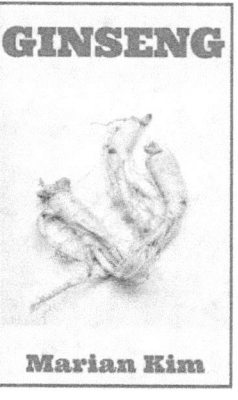

GINSENG

Marian Kim

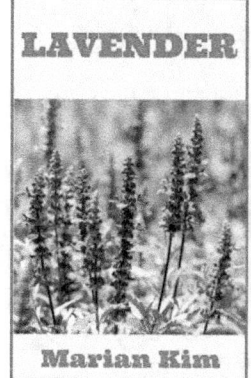

LAVENDER

Marian Kim

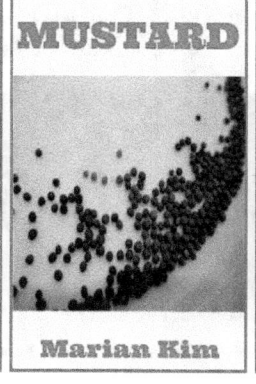

MUSTARD

Marian Kim

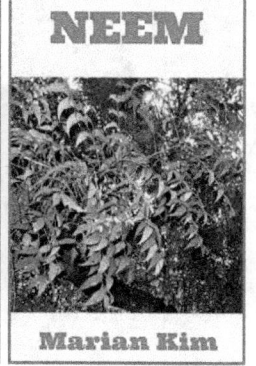

NEEM

Marian Kim

NUTMEG & MACE
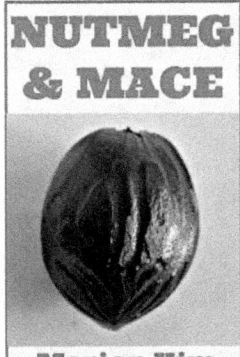
Marian Kim

OREGANO
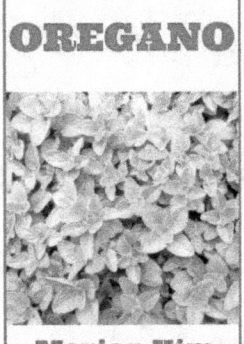
Marian Kim

PAPRIKA
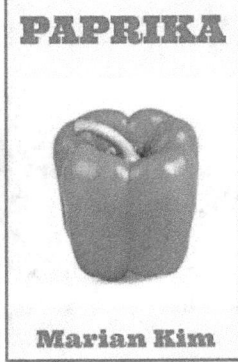
Marian Kim

PARSLEY
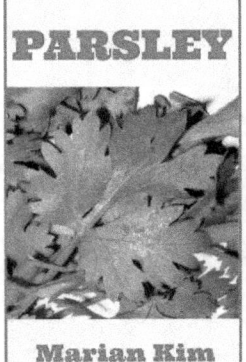
Marian Kim

BLACK & WHITE PEPPER
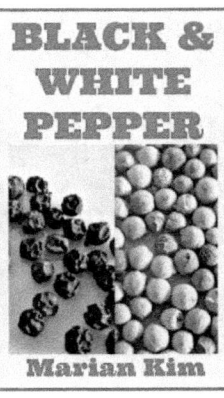
Marian Kim

PEPPERMINT
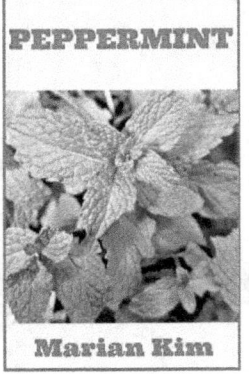
Marian Kim

ROSE HIPS
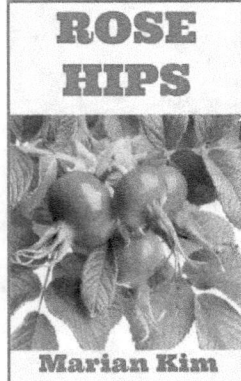
Marian Kim

ROSE PETALS
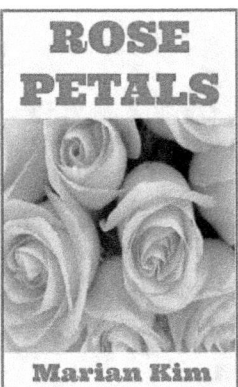
Marian Kim

ROSEMARY
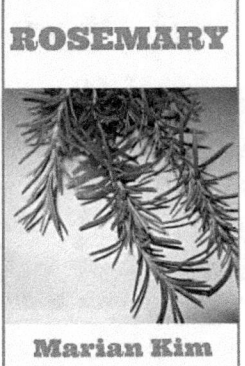
Marian Kim

SAGE

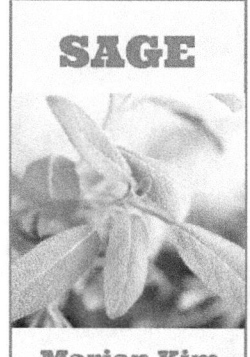

Marian Kim

ST. JOHN'S WORT

Marian Kim

STAR ANISE

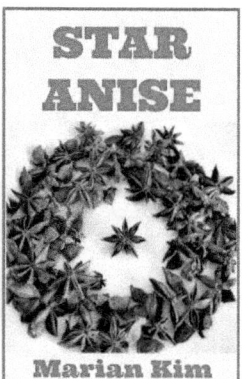

Marian Kim

STINGING NETTLE

Marian Kim

THYME

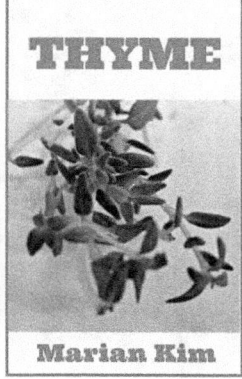

Marian Kim

TURMERIC

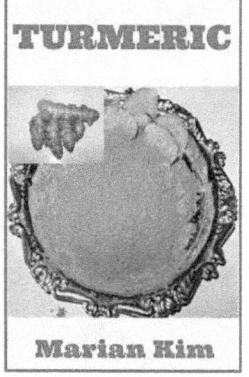

Marian Kim

WITCH HAZEL

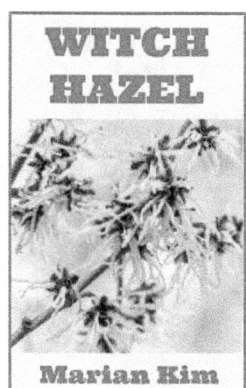

Marian Kim

YARROW

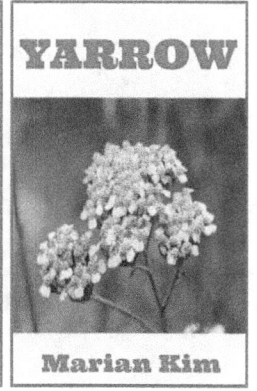

Marian Kim

*****